Eye Strain

Causes, Symptoms, Treatment, and Conditions

By Frederick Earlstein

Foreword

In the modern, connected world, eye strain afflicts us all at one time or another. Whether it's pushing to make a deadline at work or just spending too much time squinting at our cell phones, we overtax our eyes on a daily basis.

The minimal amount of time on a computer to cause computer vision syndrome is just two hours per day. I don't know about you, but I put in that much time before my second cup of coffee every day!

While eye strain is not dangerous, the burning, itching, gritty feeling accompanied by blurred vision and difficulty focusing is exhausting and negatively effects productivity.

Regardless of whether we are placing the blame on the computer or the more traditional "reading too much," it's easy to wear your eyes out. (For the record, I don't think you can *ever* read too much.)

With practical steps to change your work environment and to take better care of your eyes, eye strain can be easily improved or prevented completely.

It is imperative, however, to make sure that your eyes are healthy and that you do not need corrective lenses, or that the lenses that you are wearing do not need to be updated. The first step in solving chronic eye strain is a visit to the eye doctor for a comprehensive exam.

In the following pages, I will break down the basic

information about what causes eye strain, explain normal visual irregularities, and suggest simple methods to give your eyes the break they need and deserve.

The good news is that once you acknowledge eye strain as a problem, getting on top of the issue typically requires only minimal, common sense changes to your habits and working environment.

Acknowledgments

I would like to express my gratitude towards my family, friends, and colleagues for their kind co-operation and encouragement which helped me in completion of this book.

My thanks and appreciations go to my colleagues and people who have willingly helped me out with their abilities.

Table of Contents

Chapter 1 - The Problem of Eye Strain

None of us are immune to the effects of eye strain, nor is it possible to completely avoid the phenomenon. Every graduate student knows the feeling of reading until the words blur on the page.

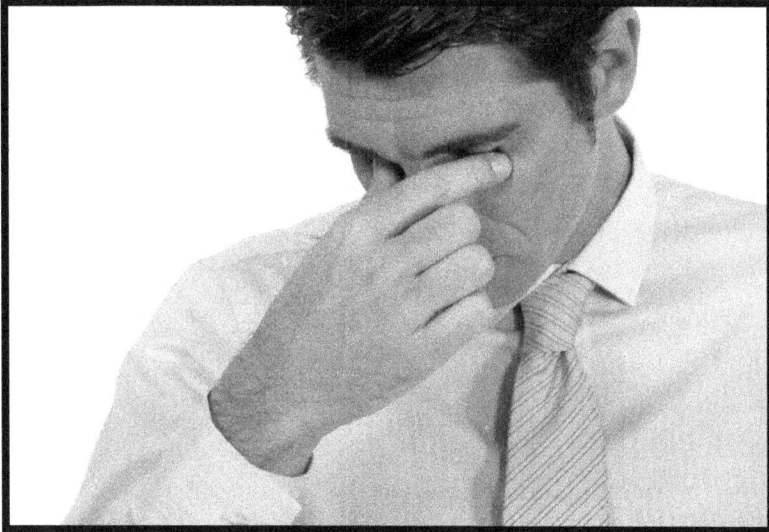

New parents know the way their eyes feel after a sleepless night of walking the floor with a crying baby. And anyone who has traveled can attest to the effects of several hours in an airplane cockpit full of stale, recirculated air. The human eyes are sensitive structures, ones on which we rely heavily, and ones we often abuse with impunity.

What is Eye Strain?

Eye strain or fatigue is a common complaint, one that is more annoying than serious, but that can compromise our ability to work effectively while increasing an overall sense of being tired and over worked. The scientific name for the condition is asthenopia.

Generally the problem can be improved and prevented altogether by common sense measures. If, however, eye fatigue is a persistent problem with headaches, discomfort, double vision, or any other changes in your sight, consult an eye doctor immediately.

Although we all rely heavily on our vision, most of us have no understanding of how our eyes work or how our brains interpret the visual signals they receive.

The Anatomy of the Eye

In order to understand the structure of the eye, let's follow the path that light takes as it enters the eyeball. First light passes through the clear layer at the front of the structure called the **cornea**, a space filled with a watery liquid that helps the eyeball maintain its shape.

The fluid, called the **aqueous humor**, sits in place around the colored portion of the eye known as the **iris**. The opening at the center of the iris is called the **pupil**. The pupil expands and contracts according to the amount of available light.

Light passes through this opening, which appears as a black dot and next reaches a round, clear **lens**. A tiny muscle encircles the lens, bending it as necessary to allow for both near and far vision.

At the back of the eye there are three layers: the **sclera**, the **choroid**, and the **retina**. The sclera is the white part of the eye that protects the eyeball. The choroid is the middle layer. The inner layer or retina is comprised of nerve endings that translate light into signals comprehensible to the brain.

The gelatin-like substance that fills the back of the eyeball and defines its round shape is called the **vitreous humor**. At the rear of all of these structures lies the **optic nerve**, which transmits signals from the retina to the brain where they are interpreted as visual input.

Each eye is moved by the coordination of six muscles so that you can continue to look at something even if you move your head. Four of these pull the eyeball into a straight line up, down, or to the side, while two rotate or turn the eye.

Like all the parts of the human body, the eyes are subject to fatigue from overuse. Since we rely so heavily on our vision in our day-to-day lives, eye strain can not only wear us out, it can affect our productivity and our enjoyment of many "time off" activities.

We rely on varying levels of eye care professionals to help us keep our eyes healthy and to provide treatments and corrective lenses to improve and stabilize our vision.

Eye Care Professionals

There are three types of eye care professionals each with a

different level of accreditation and skill:

- **Optician** - Opticians assemble, fit, and sell prescription eyeglasses and, subject to specific state regulations, potentially contact lenses as well.

- **Optometrists** - An individual who holds a degree in optometry is a doctor and has been trained not only to evaluate the degree of a person's vision and correct abnormalities with an eyeglass prescription, but also to diagnose general eye conditions.

- **Ophthalmologist** - An ophthalmologist holds either a degree as a Doctor of Osteopathy or as a Doctor of Medicine. These professionals provide comprehensive care, evaluating the health of the eyes, prescribing corrective lenses, diagnosing and treating common and complex eye problems, and performing eye surgeries.

What then, are the most common causes of eye strain or fatigue?

Causes of Eye Strain

Any activity that requires concentrated use of the eyes for a long period of time can cause eye fatigue. Common culprits include reading, writing, and driving, but you can also wear your eyes out squinting in bright sunlight and struggling to see in dim light.

The digital age has introduced many visually exhausting

tasks in which we engage on a daily basis including staring at the screen of a computer, checking emails and webpages on our smartphones, and playing endless hours of video games.

Computer Vision Syndrome

The prevalence of computers in our daily lives has led to a completely separate definition of eye fatigue from this source. It is estimated that as many as 10 million eye examinations per year are prompted by computer vision syndrome, which affects 50% to 90% of computer workers in the United States.

Researchers have determined that we hold our digital devices much closer to our eyes than we would books or newspapers, which forces our eyes to work harder focusing on tiny type.

Humans also blink less than the normal 18 times per minute when they look at a computer screen, so their eyes are not refreshed as often. This causes dry, burning eyes that are not only tired, but also itchy.

Symptoms of Eye Strain

The symptoms of eye fatigue decrease a person's productivity level and are made worse if sleep deprivation is a factor. During sleep, essential nutrients are returned to the eyes. The less sleep an individual gets, the more irritated their eyes will be. If you have eye strain, you may experience:

- soreness
- redness and irritation
- difficulty focusing
- blurred and/or double vision
- dry or watery eyes
- light sensitivity

It is also common to feel pain and tension in the neck, shoulders, and back with a case of eye strain.

Any time you think you may be suffering from eye strain, it's generally a good idea to get a comprehensive eye exam, especially if it's been quite a while since you've seen the eye doctor.

Chapter 2 – Eye Strain and Associated Problems

Like any common condition, there's a great deal of misinformation about eye strain that circulates as "common knowledge."

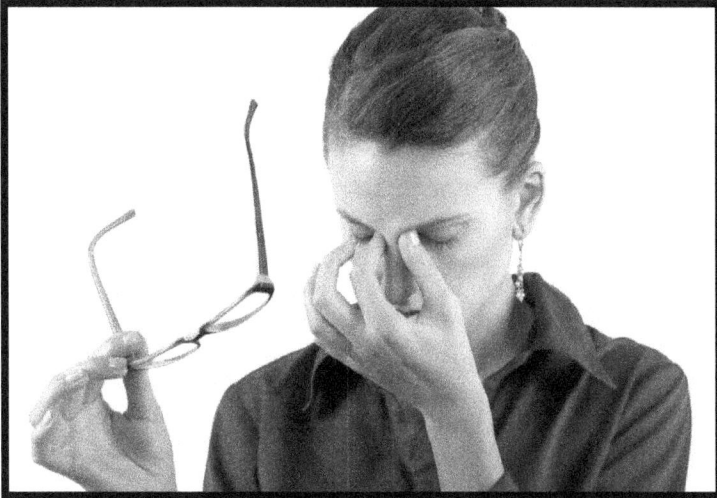

Is there a relationship between "floaters" and eye fatigue?

If your eyes are tired are you risking retinal detachment?

Do you have to be sensitive to light to suffer from eye strain?

Are dry eyes and eye fatigue the same thing?

What's the connection with eye strain and migraines?

To understand more about these associated problems, real or imagined, let's look at each one in turn.

Does Eye Strain Cause "Floaters?"

It is a myth that eye strain causes floaters. These anomalies are pieces of the vitreous of the eye that have broken loose. The fibers may appear as spots, flecks, specks, or even cobwebs. They float around the eye and until we really focus on them or we are looking at the white screen of a computer, they are not annoying or troublesome.

Eye strain is not responsible for the formation of floaters. At birth, the vitreous of the eye has a gel-like consistency, but as we age that changes.

Floaters naturally get worse over time. The only time that floaters should be considered a potential medical emergency is if you see a shower of these spots accompanied by flashes of light. This could indicate a retinal tear or detachment. In this instance, you should seek immediate medical attention.

Retinal Detachment

Retinal detachment occurs when the retina becomes separated from the underlying choroid tissue causing a loss of vision in the affected area. It is a serious condition that, if left untreated, can cause a permanent loss of vision.

Risk factors for retinal detachment include:

- being extremely nearsighted
- suffering an eye injury
- cataract surgery

- family history of retinal detachment

A retinal tear may be a precursor to an actual retinal detachment. Fluid passing through the tear can cause the retina to separate from the underlying tissue. Detachments may happen with no warning, but a retinal tear can be signaled by warning flashes of light and a cascade of floaters.

When the retina has become fully detached, you will not only see flashes of light and floaters, but your peripheral vision will darken. It is imperative that you seek medical attention immediately. The doctor will dilate your eyes in order to view the retina clearly.

There are several ways to treat a detached retina. Some, like laser or cryopexy (freezing), can repair a tear before it progresses to a full detachment. Others, like the scleral buckle, involve supporting the total structure of the eye until the tear heals. The approach will vary in each case.

Retinal detachments can be prevented with regular eye exams and a healthy lifestyle, including proper maintenance of diabetes and high blood pressure. You should also wear appropriate eye protection during sports activities and when working with chemicals and tools.

Although it is extremely rare for eye strain to result in a retinal detachment, your eyes are in a weakened condition when fatigued and thus more vulnerable to all manner of injuries and irritations.

Photophobia and Eyestrain

Photophobia is extreme sensitivity to light of all kinds including indoor and outdoor sources with a range of accompanying symptoms. This is a special sub-category of eye strain, since the fatigue from photophobia can feel like a physical assault.

Symptoms of photophobia include:

- severe eye strain
- crushing fatigue
- drowsiness
- nausea
- dizziness
- anxiety
- irritability
- discomfort

Photophobia can easily trigger severe headaches or outright migraines. This condition may be genetic or the result of an injury like a concussion, a traumatic brain injury, whiplash, or some other underlying medical condition. The brain literally cannot adjust to varying levels of brightness in the environment. People with light-colored eyes are more susceptible to photophobia.

Sunglasses are not sufficient to provide comfort and protection from all forms of lighting. Sufferers may require glasses with special filters to function on a daily basis, and must wear the glasses at all times.

Dry Eye Syndrome and Eye Strain

Dry eye syndrome is also called keratoconjunctivitis sicca. It is a disease of the eye that causes insufficient production of lubricating tears. Women are more likely to develop this condition than men and it is increasingly common as we age.

Symptoms include:

- burning and irritation
- a gritty sensation of having something in the eye
- blurred vision
- severe eye strain

Artificial tears must be used on a regular basis to relieve the discomfort and fatigue.

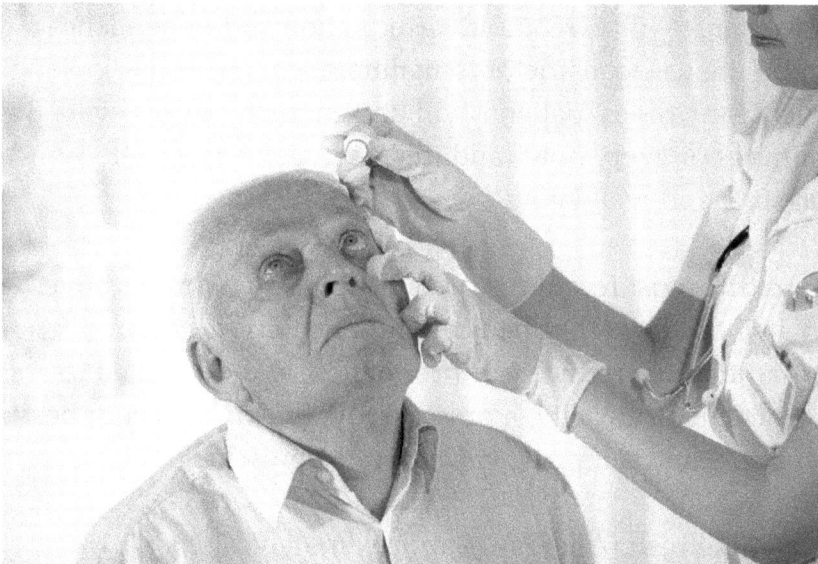

Selecting Artificial Tears

Although artificial tear products are most often suggested as a solution for dry eye, they are also a powerful tool to use to lessen the effects of all types of eye strain. There are, however, so many choices of these over-the-counter products that picking the "best" one is a difficult proposition.

In an article for *Review of Ophthalmology*, "OTC Drops: Telling the Tears Apart" by Michelle Stephenson (October 2012), John Sheppard, MD, a professor of ophthalmology, microbiology, and molecular biology at Eastern Virginia Medical School defined the problem this way:

"Invariably, when patients bring in their drops, they will be the Wal-Mart or Safeway brand of tears, which are by far the most inferior tears on the market. Or, worse yet, they will use a topical vasoconstrictor like Visine, which induces vascular fragility, rebound vasodilation and dependence upon the vasoconstrictor to maintain a quiet, white-looking eye. Many times, patients will present using drops every 30 minutes or every hour, and this has a deleterious effect on lifestyle and well-being."

Since the most recent research indicates that preservatives in artificial tears, like benzalkonium chloride, cause inflammation, reduce tear production, and are linked to corneal neurotoxicity, a preservative-free drop is your best choice. Stand out products in this category include

- Refresh (Allergan) - approximately $30 per 2.17 ounces

- TheraTears - approximately $12 per 1 ounce
- Soothe (Bausch & Lomb) - approximately $11 per 0.5 ounces
- Systane (Alcon) - approximately $15 per 1 ounce

Although these products are more expensive than more generic options, they have an excellent reputation among eye care professionals. If you need to use lubricating drops more than four times per day, you should choose a preservative-free solution.

Migraine Headaches and Vision

Anyone who has experienced the pain of a migraine headache knows that visual symptoms are part of the experience. Migraine sufferers often see flashing spots, wavy lines, and may even experience temporary blindness.

A specific type of visual incident called a retinal or ocular migraine is caused by the same underlying inflammatory substances that trigger a normal migraine, but there is no accompanying pain.

The first experience of an ocular migraine is still frightening, however. Typically the episode begins when a small blind spot or scotoma appears in the central lines of vision.

As you become more aware of its presence, you'll see flickering wavy lines or scintillations on the borders of the spot. At this point the scotoma may move across your field of vision making it impossible for you to see what you're doing with any degree of accuracy.

Take all the necessary precautions to ensure your safety and that of those around you. If you are driving, pull over until the incident passes. Otherwise, simply relax wherever you may be and wait until your vision returns to normal.

If you have never had an ocular migraine before, consider having a comprehensive eye exam to rule out any underlying physical cause like a detached retina.

The entire episode will likely last no more than 30 minutes. Ocular migraines are harmless in nature and may affect one or both eyes. Such an event is not tied to eye strain any more than a normal migraine, but is the result of a release of chemicals deep in the brain.

Researchers estimate that 70% of people who suffer from migraines of any type have a genetic basis for the disorder.

Eye Strain and Allergies

Seasonal and environmental allergies have a significant impact on the eyes, including itching and burning that leads to almost non-stop rubbing, at which point the eyes either become dry, gritty, and uncomfortable, or they start to tear and run profusely. Other symptoms may include:

- swelling of the lids
- swelling of the surrounding tissues
- redness and irritation
- light sensitivity

Allergic symptoms are not just annoying, they may also render the person incapable of engaging in outdoor activities or playing with pets. Because your eyes are fighting off so many symptoms at once, fatigue is a natural consequence of the stress.

Allergens effect the eyes the same way they do other parts of the body, causing the release of histamine and other chemicals that dilate the blood vessels, cause the mucous membranes to itch, and lead to inflammation of the surrounding tissues.

For seasonal allergies, the best solution may be staying indoors, while many environmental triggers, like mold and dust mites can be removed or minimized. It is important not to use eye drops that will further dry out the eyes, so consult your ophthalmologist or allergy specialist to help you choose the correct product.

Do *not* rub your eyes! Use hold or cold compresses to help alleviate the itchy, gritty feeling. The more you rub your eyes, the greater chance you have of introducing bacteria and other contaminants that may lead to an actual infection rather than an allergic reaction.

Conjunctivitis

Conjunctivitis or pink eye is an inflammation of the thin, clear tissue covering the white part of the eye and the inside of the eyelid. This tissue, called the conjunctiva, may become irritated by the presence of a virus or bacteria, or due to exposure to chemical irritants (chlorine, smoke, shampoo). Allergens such as dust and pollen can also be involved.

Conjunctivitis is contagious, but it is not a serious health risk unless it occurs in newborn babies, where the inflammation may threaten the child's vision. The major symptoms include:

- redness in the white of the eye and inner eyelid
- excessive tearing
- crusty, yellow discharge on the eyelashes, especially upon awakening
- green or white discharge
- itching and burning
- blurred vision
- increased light sensitivity

The doctor will use a cotton swab to collect a sample of the discharge from your eye for analysis to identify the bacteria or virus involved. If a form of bacteria is the problem, antibiotics, either as drops, ointments, or pills will be prescribed. The infection should improve within a week. For a viral cause, the infection will have to run its course.

The viral form of conjunctivitis is highly contagious. Always wash your hands frequently and avoid contact with others. Throw away any contacts you've worn during the infection. (Women should also discard all eye makeup.)

Again, conjunctivitis is not caused by eye strain, but if you are rubbing your eyes a great deal due to eye fatigue, it's extremely easy to introduce bacteria or viruses into your eyes, thus triggering an infection.

Sties

A hordeolum or sty is a painful, red lump that sits at the edge of your eyelid. It has the appearance of a small pimple or boil. It is not uncommon for pus to be present. Although the lesion is typically outside the eyelid it can form on the inner portion of the lid as well.

Over a period of several days, a sty could resolve on its own. Apply a warm washcloth to the eyelid several times a day for 10-15 minutes to relieve the discomfort and to help the pus in the sty to release on its own. Do not be alarmed if your eyelid swells, or if you see tearing and crust in the eye.

If, however, the sty is not improving within 48 hours or the swelling extends beyond the eyelid, you may want to consult your doctor.

Sties are caused by bacteria that comes into contact with your eyes when you rub or touch your eyes without washing your hands. The main culprit is *bacterium staphylococcus.*

People who wear contact lenses are at high risk. Do not put your lenses in place without washing your hands first, and always disinfect your lenses before you put them in. Also, women should not leave their eye makeup on overnight or use cosmetics that are old or that have expired.

Sties are not a cause of eye fatigue, but the lesions are so uncomfortable they can make an existing case of eye fatigue worse.

Twitching Eyes

Twitches and ticks or spasms in the eye are fairly common, typically involving the lower lid only. Although most episodes are of a short duration, a twitch can occasionally last for days or even weeks. The condition may be due to any one of the following factors:

- stress
- fatigue
- eye strain
- caffeine
- alcohol
- dry eyes
- nutritional deficiencies
- allergies

Therefore, twitching eyes are a result of eye strain, not a cause of the condition. Although incredibly annoying, twitching is a benign phenomenon. Your best options are to lay off the caffeine, give your eyes the rest they need, and ignore the twitching. The more you think about it, the worse it will get!

As is always the case, if the problem becomes chronic, or lasts for several days, see your eye doctor. There are rare neurological conditions that can present with twitching of the eyelids, but only your physician can make that determination.

Eye Strain and Ptosis

A ptosis is an upper or lower eyelid that droops because the muscles that raise the eyelid are abnormally weak. Some individuals are born with the condition, while others experience the drooping as they age or as a symptom of another illness.

The degree to which the eyelid droops may vary considerably. Some cases are slight, while in more serious instances the lid covers the pupil entirely. A ptosis is not the same thing as a lazy eye or wandering eye (amblyopia.) Although the eye affected by the ptosis may be weaker in terms of visual acuity and is more prone to astigmatism, it still tracks appropriately.

Although there are surgical remedies for a ptosis, the vast majority of people with the drooping opt to leave it alone. As a possible post-surgical complication, the eye might lose the ability to close completely, necessitating the use of lubricating drops for life.

Having a ptosis does not make a person more susceptible to eye strain, although the affected eye will be more likely to simply close when the individual doesn't feel well, is extremely tired, or is subject to harsh lighting. This can affect a person's binocular and weaken their depth perception.

Persistent Eye Strain

If none of the usual countermeasures help to relieve your

eye strain, get a medical evaluation. You may need glasses, or the prescription you are using may be out of date. You could also have an underlying condition that is causing your eye muscles to be out of balance.

Most people go years without replacing their eyeglasses, not realizing that even subtle changes in your prescription may be working against you. It's possible that you may be straining to see without even realizing it.

Some signs that you may need new glasses include:

- frequent headaches
- neck aches
- frequent squinting

You may need "occupation specific" glasses to help you keep your eyes well rested. Many people now avail themselves of computer glasses with a focal range specifically calibrated for the distance from their eyes to their monitors.

Some people also benefit from using a slight gray or brown tint in their lenses to help reduce their sensitivity to light. The technology behind eyewear and corrective lenses is constantly evolving and improving. Talk to your eye doctor. You may have more options than you realize.

Chapter 3 – Working With Eye Care Professionals

Putting off going to the eye doctor is an easy thing to do. Eyeglasses are expensive. No one likes waiting for a new prescription to be ready or getting used to a new pair of frames. We tell ourselves that we can see just fine even though the prescription we're using is 3 or 4 years old and our eyes seem to be tired all the time. One of the best ways to save yourself from eye strain is to simply see your eye doctor every year!

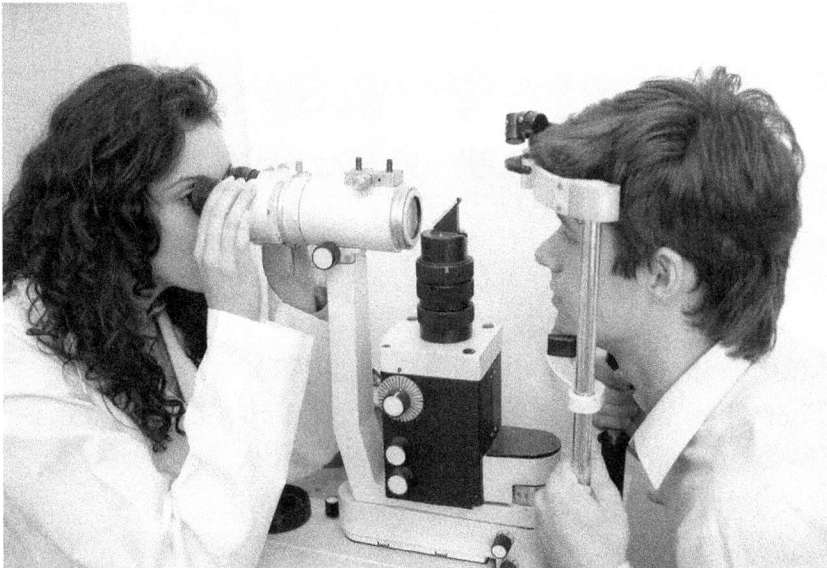

Comprehensive Eye Exams

A comprehensive eye exam will look for a range of visual and physical problems using a battery of standard tests. Such annual checkups are not just for individuals who wear glasses and require an adjustment in their prescription, but should also be a part of a complete program of preventive healthcare.

Annual testing is critical for the early detection and treatment of:

- glaucoma
- age-related macular degeneration
- cataracts
- diabetic retinopathy

Children should have their vision checked at 6 months, age 3, and just before they enter the first grade.

Adults should have their eyes checked every two years at minimum and annually after the age of 60. If you suffer from diabetes or high blood pressure, or if your work is visually demanding, more frequent check-ups may be indicated.

Most visits to the eye doctor take half an hour to an hour. There's nothing to be worried or fearful about. Eye exams don't hurt, and most people actually find the experience interesting.

What to Expect During an Eye Exam

During your visit to the eye doctor, you will be asked a series of questions about your medical history, work, and lifestyle to determine how you use your eyes and if any other health problems you have had in the past or may be experiencing currently could be affecting your eyes.

Expect to provide a list of medications used and to give a description of the environmental conditions you encounter most frequently.

The standard tests performed during the exam will include:

- **eye muscle movement** - This allows the doctor to check the alignment of the eyes as well as your ability to visually track objects in different directions.

- **cover test** - While you look at a distant object, the doctor will cover and uncover each eye in turn to independently observe movement and tracking.

- **external exam / pupillary reaction** - This test judges the reaction of the pupils to light and objects at a close distance. The doctor will also examine the exterior of the eye including the position of the eyelids and the condition of the whites of the eye.

- **visual acuity test** - The visual acuity test is the one most commonly thought of as an "eye" test. You will be asked to read progressively smaller letters on a chart using both eyes and each eye individually.

- **retinoscopy** - While you look forward at the eye chart, the doctor will shine a light into your eyes and flip through lenses in a machine called a phoropter to check how light reflects from the eye. This allows the doctor to develop an approximate lens prescription.

- **refraction testing** - This is the process by which a lens prescription is refined, either by use of a computerized refractor or manually. ("Which is better? A or B?")

- **biomicroscope** - Also called the slit lamp, this device lights up and magnifies the front of the eye allowing the doctor to examine the cornea, iris, lens, and anterior chamber for signs of disease or irregularities.

- **ophthalmoscopy** - After dilating the pupils, the doctor uses an ophthalmoscope to examine the retina, retinal blood vessels, vitreous, and optic nerve head at the back of the eye.

- **glaucoma testing** - Several different methods can be used to determine the level of fluid pressure* of the eye including the tonometer, which barely touch the surface of the eye. The non-contact version of this test is the "puff of air," where pressure is measured in relation to resistance.

- **pachymetry** - A measurement of the thickness of the corneas via ultrasound. Pachymetry is frequently used for patients who may need corneal surgery.

- **pupil dilation** - The use of drops to force the pupils to become fully enlarged so the doctor may see inside the eyes more clearly. The drops make the eyes more sensitive to light and blur the vision. These effects may persist for several hours.

- **visual field test** - Also called perimetry, this test determines the size of the area in front of you that you can see without moving your eyes. It is used to map the edge of your peripheral vision.

* Normal pressure in the eye falls in a range of 12-21 mmHg. Anything above 21 mmHG is considered to be abnormal. There are no evident symptoms of glaucoma and it is not a cause of eye strain or fatigue.

A typical diagnosis will find that a person is either nearsighted or farsighted and may have some degree of astigmatism present. If these kinds of visual irregularities are not corrected with prescription lenses, eye fatigue is a natural consequence because your eyes are working overtime to compensate for the problem.

Typical Visual Irregularities

Although there are many conditions that can affect the eyes, when you go in for an eye visit, especially if you are about to receive prescription lenses for the first time, you will be diagnosed as nearsighted and/or farsighted and you may have some degree of astigmatism.

There are two parts of the eye that function together to focus our vision. The cornea transmits light into the eye, while the transparent lens focuses those rays toward the retina. Both the cornea and the lens can change shape to create precisely focused images for the retina.

If one of those elements is not evenly curved, however, the

light rays are not refracted correctly with some degree of visual distortion resulting.

Nearsightedness

Nearsightedness or myopia refers to a visual condition which limits people to seeing objects in sharp focus only when those items are nearer to the eye.

Myopia affects approximately 40% of the population. Even though many children are myopic, they may not be accurately assessed until age 20 or later.

When myopia is present, the eyeball is longer than normal, which distorts the cornea's ability to focus by causing the lens to assume an irregular shape.

Myopia can develop gradually or suddenly and may be inherited, especially if one or both parents also have the condition. However, daily use of the eyes is a more telling factor in the vast majority of cases.

People who read a great deal or spend many hours working on detailed tasks, for instance, are more susceptible to being nearsighted.

Those at the greatest risk are the professionals who spend most of their time in front of a computer screen including, but not limited to, writers, architects, graphic artists, game designers, and programmers. In these cases the condition may be "pseudo myopia" or visual stress resulting in a reduced capacity for distance vision.

Other medical conditions may cause myopia as a secondary symptom. For instance inconsistent blood sugar levels in diabetic individuals may cause myopia.

The most common symptoms of myopia include:

- headaches
- eyestrain
- squinting
- fatigue while driving or playing sports
- blinking frequently
- rubbing the eyes frequently

Although it is an extremely rare condition affecting approximately 2% of Americans, progressive degenerative myopia can lead to legal blindness. This condition may also be referred to as pathological or malignant myopia.

Farsightedness

People who are farsighted can see objects at a distance clearly, but have difficulty with things close at hand. The proper name for the condition is hyperopia, which results from a flattening of the normal curvature of the cornea. The lens cannot adjust itself to become rounder as needed to focus on near objects.

Most children are born with a degree of hyperopia that disappears as their eyes lengthen with normal growth. Paradoxically, farsightedness in children is often detected when they sit closer to, not farther away from the television and squint to try to distinguish lines and details.

This behavior is a combination of their developing brain's ability to interpret images as well as the physical defect present in the structure of the eye.

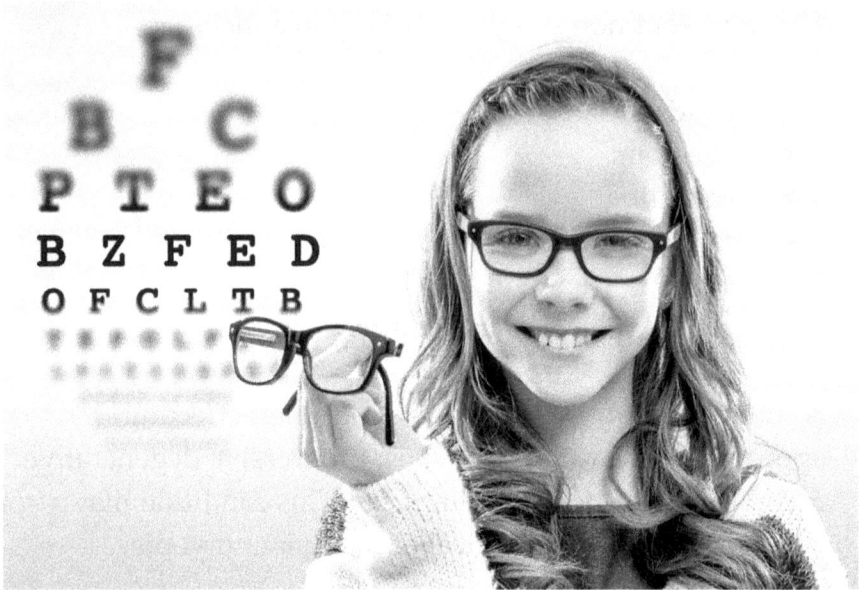

Often the first actual clue that the child is farsighted is when they cannot catch balls or other objects that are thrown to them during play activities. Some symptoms of acute and uncorrected hyperopia include:

- a burning sensation in the eyes
- aching and discomfort
- headache and fatigue

Poor performance in school may also be an indication, and in some instances when no eye exam has been performed, untreated farsightedness may even be mistaken for attention deficit hyperactivity disorder (ADHD).

Astigmatism

Astigmatism is a visual condition that causes blurred vision due to an irregularly shaped cornea or an abnormal curvature of the lens. It's perfectly normal for astigmatism to accompany near or farsightedness.

A small degree of astigmatism doesn't cause problems, but the more severe it becomes, the more the individual will suffer from distorted or blurred vision with accompanying headaches and discomfort leading to eye strain.

There are three types of astigmatism:

- myopic astigmatism
- hyperopic astigmatism
- mixed astigmatism

Each is classified as regular or irregular, a reference to the focal power of the eye's horizontal and/or vertical meridians.

Astigmatism is detected during a regular eye examination and it requires the use of prescription lenses to restore normal vision and avoid resulting eye strain.

Presbyopia

People who have never worn eyeglasses may be surprised when their near vision begins to deteriorate after age 40. This is a natural consequence of aging called presbyopia. According to the World Health Organization, more than a billion people around the world are presbyopic.

One of the first signs of presbyopia is called "playing the trombone." In order to read books, newspapers, magazines, and menus, you must hold the material at arm's length to achieve the correct focus.

Any kind of close hand work, like fine sewing or writing a letter by hand, causes eyestrain unless you are using additional magnification.

It is a myth, however, that women require reading glasses sooner than men due to a difference in their eyes. The real reason is that women's arms are, on average, shorter than men's arms and therefore they have a more difficult time holding things at arm's length.

Presbyopia is caused by a gradual hardening of the lens of the eye due to changes in the proteins present in the structure. As the lens loses it elasticity, its ability to alter its shape diminishes, making focusing harder and harder.

The most common correction for presbyopia is a prescription for bifocal or progressive lenses. Such prescriptions contain a top adjustment to aid with distance vision and a lower one to correct focus closer to the eyes.

Progressive lenses offer a more gradual transition between the two adjustments, providing a middle ground magnification as well. This type of lens has replaced the older variation called the trifocal.

For individuals who do not have astigmatism, which requires a rotational correction as well as magnification, the use of over-the-counter reading glasses is often all that is required once presbyopia is present.

Presbyopia is a progressive condition, so you will need increasingly stronger levels of magnification as you age.

What If I Can't Use OTC Readers?

People who are feeling the effects of presbyopia but who also have astigmatism can't use over-the-counter reading glasses because the lenses do not have the necessary rotational correction.

Prescription eyeglasses are expensive. If your existing prescription is working for you in the majority of situations in your life, or you simply can't afford to change it immediately, try a product called PC Peekers (www.pcpeekers.com).

The Peekers fit behind your existing lenses and alter the magnification of the prescription. Although Peekers are intended to help people see a computer screen without having to purchase additional computer "glasses," you can experiment with their effect.

I do have computer and reading glasses, but I have found that using the Peekers with those prescriptions gives me the additional boost I need to overcome my presbyopia and do really close, detailed work when I'm engaged in hobbies or working with very tiny type.

Depending on the vendor, PC Peekers are available at a price range of $18-$30.

Chapter 4 – Dealing With Eye Strain

Now that you understand more about the structure of the eye and how irregularities effect vision, you should see that dealing with eye strain is often a matter of simply managing your environment and improving your habits.

Preventing Eye Fatigue

Many simple environmental changes can lessen or completely prevent the effects of eye strain. Some of these tips for lessening eye fatigue seem unnecessary, but you will be surprised by how much they help.

Keep your computer screen clean.

For starters, pay attention to your computer screen. Keep it dust free and clean away smudges and fingerprints that reduce contrast while worsening glare and reflections.

Select screens that can be tilted and swiveled to obtain the best viewing angle, and place them 20-26 inches away from your eyes and slightly below eye level.

Go with the largest computer screen you can afford. Screens that are 19 inches and up will create less eye strain.

Use softer lighting and take steps to minimize glare.

Use lighting in your work environment that reduces glare and reflections, and make sure that your chair is adjustable. This is especially important if you cannot change the physical orientation of your computer screen.

Excessively bright light coming into your work space from outside is very tiring for the eyes. When you are working on a computer, the ambient lighting in the room should be about half as bright as the typical "norm" for most offices.

Use drapes or shades to reduce exterior light and turn off overhead fluorescent lights. Rely instead on floor lamps that provide soft incandescent or LED-based illumination.

Choose full-spectrum bulbs.

Although most of us don't realize it, light has "color." Some people find "full spectrum" bulbs that have no yellow or blue tint to be more restful since the light they emit is meant to mimic natural sunlight.

If you can't control glare any other way, look into getting an anti-glare screen for your monitor. If you're really in control of your office environment, paint the walls a darker color and opt for a matte finish.

Stay out of drafts.

If your desk or work area is in line with an air conditioning vent or fan, move yourself out of the flow of air, or block it in some way. Sitting in a current of air for long periods of time contributes to dry eyes.

That, in turn, leads to the natural reaction of reaching up to rub your eyes, which will only add to the irritation. These are the kinds of things that seriously compound eye strain and make it a chronic condition.

Take breaks and don't forget to blink!

Follow the 20-20-20 rule. Every 20 minutes look approximately 20 feet in the distance and hold your gaze there for 20 seconds. Always use glasses for the computer that have an anti-reflective coating.

Even if you have to put a sticky note on your screen that says "blink," make sure that you keep your eyes refreshed with this simple and natural action.

Also, take regular breaks from your time in front of the computer screen or other close work. You can install a software option on your system to help you remember to take some time away or to improve your computer experience.

Software to Reduce Eye Strain

There are a number of software packages aimed toward helping computer users reduce their risk of eye strain. Some popular choices include:

* **EyeLeo at EyeLeo.com** - (Windows) The package includes screen blocking each hour, eye exercises, and fully customizable parameters. The software's strict mode keeps you from skipping breaks, a must if you are dyed-in-the-wool workaholic.

- **F.lux at justgetflux.com** - (OS X, Windows, Linux, iOs) - The goal of this software is to adjust the color of your screen to the time of day. It activates at sunup, gradually tinting the screen until nightfall to negate the amount of blue light you view daily. Research indicates over exposure to blue light can have a negative effect sleep patterns.

- **Awareness at iamfutureproof.com** - (OS X, Windows) This simple software does nothing but remind you to take a break. The signal is an unobtrusive and pleasant chime from a Tibetan singing bowl. You control the length of work and break times and the volume of the chime.

If you think you can manage your breaks on your own without a program to help, simply discipline yourself to set a timer on your smartphone to signal when it's time to rest your eyes for a few minutes.

Using an Anti-Glare Screen

Anti-glare screens are designed to cut down on the amount of light reflecting off a display. Not only does reflected light contribute to eye strain, it also washes out the contrast and colors on the screen while reducing its clarity and sharpness.

One way to accomplish this effect is to use a screen with a matte finish. The rough surface scatters light, rather than allowing it to be reflected, but unfortunately, this is a two-way effect. The light coming out of the screen is also scattered, creating a blur that many people find equally distasteful.

Chemically treated smooth screens maintain clarity more effectively and are excellent in spaces where you have control over the ambient lighting, like in your home office. In a professional setting, especially one with harsh overhead lighting, the matte screen approach is likely the best avenue even with its arguable limitations.

Anti-glare screens are available for devices at all levels, including tablets and smartphones. These attach to the screens without the use of an adhesive, but they can be tricky to install. It's common for the protective covering to be difficult to align, subject to dust accumulations along the edges, and worse yet, bubbles in the surface.

Although these imperfects are typically invisible when the screen is lit, they can be glaringly obvious when the device is turned off. For many people, the option is simply too untidy and ugly. I have installed many of these screens on smartphones and tablets only to rip them off in frustration after a few days.

Thankfully such screens are inexpensive, which should allow you to explore whether they can help you manage glare in your digital world without driving you crazy in the process!

Home Remedies for Tired Eyes

When you are feeling the effects of eye fatigue, there are

some simple home remedies that can offer you quick relief

- **Apply a warm wash cloth.** Soak a wash cloth in warm water and hold it against your closed eyes. This will both soothe your discomfort and help to give your eyes more moisture.

- **Splash or apply cold water.** When your eyes feel strained and tired, splash a little cold water on your face to improve circulation and reduce puffiness and swelling. Some people find a cold compress to be more soothing than a warm one.

- **Apply tea bags.** Although regular tea bags will help eye strain, chamomile is an even better option. Steep the tea bags in hot water for 3-5 minutes. Remove the bags and allow them to cool to a comfortable temperature before placing them over your closed eyelids for 5-10 minutes.

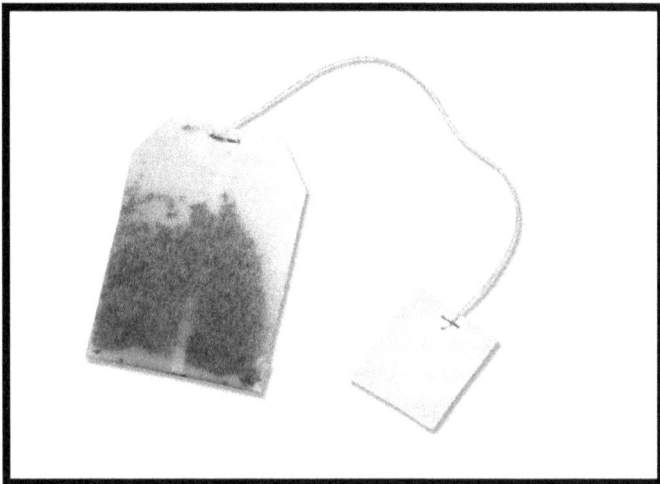

- **Use cucumber of potato compresses.** Cold slices of either cucumber or potato also offer effective relief for tired eyes. Place the vegetables in the refrigerator for at least half an hour before using. Cut thick slices to place over your eyes 1-2 times daily. Both cucumbers and potatoes have strong astringent properties that are cooling and refreshing.

- **Use artificial tears**. Artificial tears provide lubrication for your eyes, countering dryness and irritation. Use only as directed. Avoid drops that say they offer relief for red eyes. These are decongestant drops that can actually worsen the symptoms present in tired, dry eyes.

- **Improve the quality of the air around you**. A humidifier can also help, especially during the winter months and an air cleaner to take dust particles out of the air is also a good idea.

- **Gently massage your eyes 1-2 times a day**. Use your fingers to massage your eyelids and the muscles above your eyebrows for 10-20 seconds. Repeat this on the lower eyelid against the bone for 10-20 seconds. Also massage the temple and the upper cheek bones.

- **"Palm" your eyes.** This simple action creates a restful state for your eyes. Sitting upright, rub your hands together to warm them. Close your eyes and place your palms over them without applying pressure. Just enjoy the darkness for approximately

30 seconds. Repeat this technique 3-5 times a day.

Perform simple exercises. Regular eye exercises improve blood circulation and keep the eye muscles flexible. Hold a pencil or pen away from your body at arm's length. Focus on the object and bring it closer to you, maintaining your focus for as long as possible. Then move the object away again.

Bad Habits for Your Eyes

We all have habits that are not only bad for our eyes in terms of their appearance, but also in how they feel. Some behaviors to avoid include:

- **Rubbing your eyes**. The skin surrounding the eyes is one of the first areas of the skin to show aging. The more you rub your eyes, the more the tiny blood vessels just under the surface break, leading to the formation of dark circles, puffiness, drooping eyelids, and premature crow's feet.

- **Not wearing sunglasses**. Even if you don't think you need your shades, put them on! Exposing your eyes and eyelids to UV and high-energy visible (HEV) rays increases your risk for cataracts and macular degeneration. Sometimes overcast days are the worst, so don't neglect to wear good quality dark lenses that block 100% of UV rays.

- **Smoking**. There are, of course, many reasons why giving up smoking is your best health option, but smoking also increases your risk of cataracts, macular degeneration, uveitis, diabetic retinopathy, and dry eyes. Statistics indicate that smokers are four times more likely than non-smokers to experience partial or total blindness.

- **Eating a poor diet**. Without question, the American diet is a disaster, with a heavy emphasis on fast foods. Eat more fruits and vegetables to get a good mix of vitamins, minerals, and essential fatty acids. Make sure you eat plenty of leafy greens and wild-caught fish like salmon.

- **Failing to get enough sleep**. Sleep deprivation not only slows you down and ruins your concentration, you wake up with bloodshot, red eyes that are dry and often blurry. If you aren't suffering from eye strain already, sleep deprivation immediately increases your risk of suffering from tired eyes.

- **Dehydration**. Just like a poor diet, Americans are also chronically dehydrated. The recommended minimum daily consumption of water is eight glasses, but if your diet is high in sodium, you'll need more. When you're dehydrated, you experience the same eye-related symptoms typical of sleep deprivation and eye strain: dry eyes, redness, and puffy eyelids.

By improving your management of these key behaviors, you put your eyes in a far stronger position to successfully meet the demand when you do need them to work longer and harder to meet some specific goal.

Chapter 5 – Technology And Your Eyes

Although it is a myth that sitting too close to the television or computer screen will harm your eyes, we do place unusual demands on our vision with the array of digital devices that are now commonplace in our world. This is not just confined to computers, but also extends to ereaders, tablets, and smartphones.

Digital Devices and Eye Strain

In 2013, Nielsen's Digital Consumer Report found that 65% of Americans owned a smartphone, up from 44% in 2011. Smartphones were more common than digital cable (54%) and game consoles (46%).

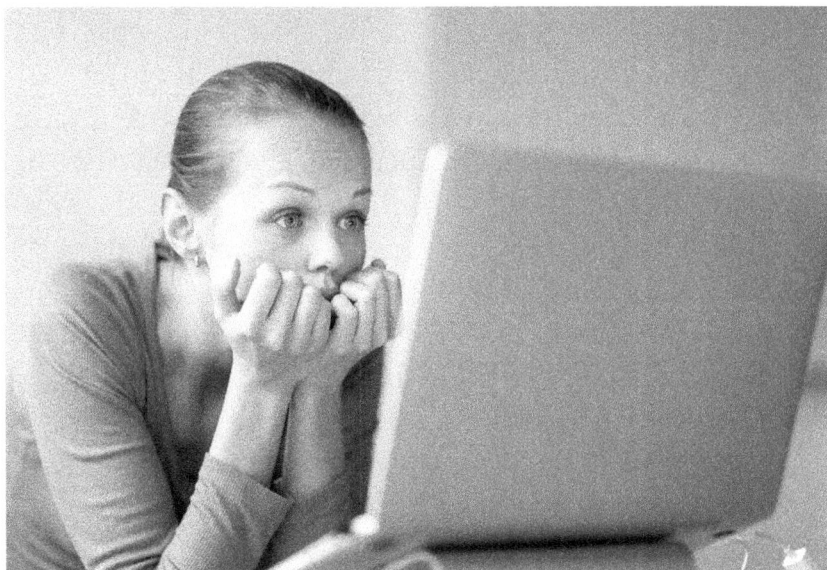

At the time, the average person owned and used at least four devices, spending at minimum 34 hours per month looking at mobile apps and browsers as compared to 27 hours at a conventional desktop computer.

Jump to January 2014, and the numbers, as reflected in Pew's Internet Project, escalated sharply.

- 90% of Americans own a cell phone of some kind
- 64% of adults own a smartphone
- 32% of adults own an e-reader
- 42% own a tablet computer

Approximately 7% of adults use their smartphone exclusively to access the Internet, while some 34% mostly use their phones for this reason.

Eye Strain and E-Readers

Many of us as children heard the admonition not to sit too close to the TV, yet today we always seem to have our faces poked in some digital device including the increasingly popular ereaders.

In an article for *The New York Times* "Bits" blog, "Do E-Readers Cause Eye Strain" by Nick Bilton in February 2010, the chair of the University of North Carolina's ophthalmology department said:

"Most of what our mothers told us about our eyes was wrong. Sitting close to a television, or computer screen, isn't bad for our eyes. It's a variety of other factors that can cause physical fatigue."

Researchers have determined that poor quality paper, like that used for newspapers and many softcover books, offers an inferior reading experience for the eyes when compared to electronic reading devices.

The screens used for various reading devices range from the E-Ink technology incorporated into the lower end Amazon Kindle line of devices to the high resolution screens with which the latest generation Apple iPads are outfitted.

The quality of the viewing experience with the devices varies by environment. E-Ink screens are exceptionally good in direct sunlight where an iPad screen might offer too much glare or be overwhelmed by the strength of the direct, ambient light.

On the other end of the spectrum, however, E-Ink can fatigue the eyes in low light because it offers less contrast. Additionally, many of these less expensive devices do not have screens with backlighting.

Professor Alan Hedge, the director of Cornell University's Human Factors and Ergonomic Laboratory, was interviewed for the same *New York Times* article. "While you're reading, your eyes make about 10,000 movements an hour," he said. "It's important to take a step back every 20 minutes and let your eyes rest."

Thankfully the current screens on all devices from ereaders to desktop machines are worlds better than the old displays where the refresh rate was so slow, a visible flicker was easily detected.

Carl Taussig, the director of the Information Surfaces Lab at Hewlett-Packard, told *The New York Times* that modern screens refresh more quickly than the human eye can see. "Today's screens update every eight milliseconds, whereas the human eye is moving at a speed between 10 and 30 milliseconds."

As is the case with most reading situations, posture and viewing position wind up being the most critical factors with ereader use. It's important when reading anything, including a traditional book, not to bend the head down for long periods of time without stretching. In this position, the neck muscles cramp, causing even more discomfort than eye strain alone.

Eyestrain and Smartphones

Your smartphone is likely causing you more eyestrain than your e-reader. The Pew Internet Project found that in 2014, approximately 67% of smartphone owners check their phones for calls, alerts, and messages even when the device has not emitted a signal for them to do so.

- 44% of users sleep with their phone next to the bed and check it during the night
- 29% say they cannot imagine living without their smartphone

The highest concentration of use by age group was in the 18-29 range, but the 30-49 age set was only 1 percentage point behind at 97% device ownership. Of Americans age 50-64, some 88% owned a cell phone, with smartphone ownership sharply on the rise.

A breakdown of specific activities on smartphones helps to explain why the time spent squinting at the small screens, which are often set an overly bright level in a darkened room, creates eye strain:

- 81% - send/receive text messages
- 60% - access the Internet
- 52% - send/receive email
- 50% - download apps
- 49% - get directions and or recommendations
- 48% - listen to music
- 21% - participate in a video call
- 8% - check in/share location via social media

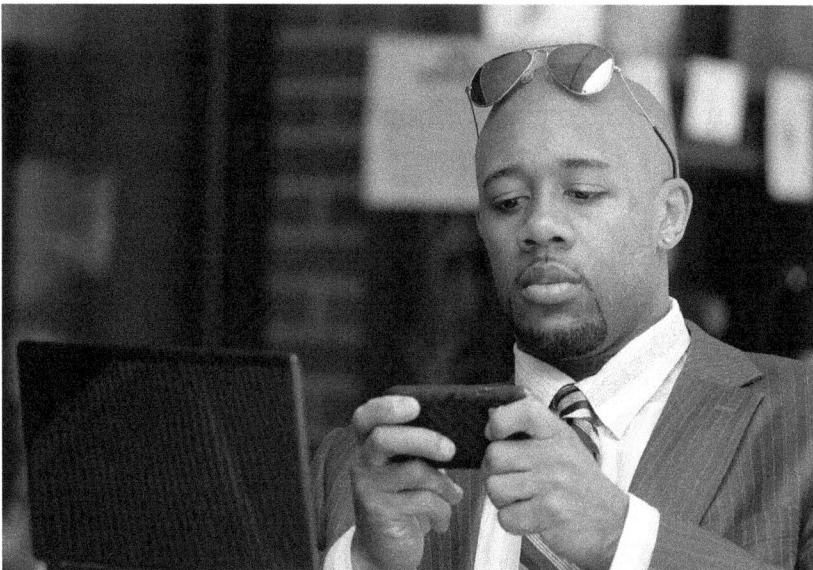

Many of the same eye-saving techniques mentioned for computer use also apply to your smartphone.

- Remember to blink to keep your eyes moist.
- Take frequent breaks following the 20-20-20 rule.
- Adjust your screen brightness.
- Keep the screen of your device clean.
- Hold the device farther away.

There are, however, some smartphone-specific steps you can take as well.

- Use a matte screen protector unless your smartphone is already equipped with anti-glare glass.

- If you check your smartphone in the night, be sure to turn the screen brightness down to minimum before you go to bed.

- Most people hold their phones about 8 inches from their face. Try to position the device at least 16-18 inches away.

If you can't see your smartphone at that distance, part of your eye strain problem may well be that you need glasses or stronger lenses in the glasses you're already wearing!

Chapter 6 - Frequently Asked Questions

Although much of this material is covered in the main text, the following frequently asked questions are meant as a quick reference source.

What is eye strain?

Eye strain is a group of uncomfortable visual symptoms associated with over use of the eyes typically from extended work requiring long periods of concentration or in poor lighting conditions. This can include, but is certainly not limited to, the use of digital devices, reading, and long periods of driving.

Is eye strain serious?

Typically eye strain is not serious and goes away when the eyes are no longer under stress. However, if your work requires you to perform functions that are hard on your eyes, you should learn the correct techniques to prevent or minimize eye strain to increase your productivity while protecting your eyes.

If I have eye strain, do I need glasses?

Not necessarily, but it is a possibility. Uncorrected vision is often a cause of eye strain, so your first step in addressing chronically fatigued eyes should be a visit to the eye doctor for a comprehensive exam. You may not need glasses all the time, but could benefit from computer or reading glasses. Also, by visiting your eye doctor, you can rule out any underlying conditions that might be overtaxing your eyes.

What are some home remedies for eye strain?

It's important to take breaks from highly concentrated work. During those times, you can apply hot or cold compresses to your eyes, lightly massage your eyes and the surrounding area, cover your eyes with the palms of your hands to create relaxing darkness, or even place warm teabags over the lids for a few minutes. For more tips on home remedies for eyestrain, see the applicable secion in the main text.

Does eye strain get worse with age?

After a fashion, yes. As we age, our eyes become less flexible and more subject to fatigue. It's also normal, after age 40, to develop presbyopia, an inability to focus clearly on objects close at hand. Even people who wear prescription lenses may find themselves reaching for a magnifying glass. The worse your vision becomes with age, the more likely your eyes will be to become fatigued with any intense visual activity.

What are the symptoms of computer vision syndrome?

Computer vision syndrome can affect anyone who uses a computer more than two hours per day. The typical symptoms include: headaches, burning eyes, fatigue, red eyes, inability to focus, blurred vision, eye twitching, and pain in the neck and shoulders.

What causes computer vision syndrome?

Our eyes react differently to words on a printed page and those on a computer screen. The edges of the characters have less definition and contrast on the computer screen, which makes it harder for our eyes to maintain sharp focus.

The eyes want to drift to a lesser level of focus called a "resting point of accommodation," and then must strain to regain focus when we are trying to pay close attention to the material on the screen. The result is eye fatigue.

Does lighting and glare effect eye strain?

Correct lighting plays a major role in managing eye strain. There should be as little outside light coming into your workplace as possible, especially if you are using a computer.

Turn off the overhead lights, and use floor lights if possible outfitted with full spectrum or LED bulbs. Minimize glare on the screen even if you have to use a screen cover or rearrange the furniture. Don't rule out the possibility of using tinted computer glasses.

Do tinted computer glasses reduce eye strain?

Yes, computer glasses with a slight brown tint will help to lessen the effects of eye strain, especially if you work in a brightly lit office where you cannot make changes to lower the light level and to reduce glare.

Can't I just use my reading glasses on the computer?

Reading glasses don't work well as computer glasses because they have been optimized to help you focus at a distance of 14-16 inches away from your eyes. Ideally, a computer screen should be 20-24 inches from your eyes.

Is it true that wearing computer glasses will make my eyes worse?

Not at all! That's a complete myth. In fact, wearing computer glasses will help prevent eye strain and protect your eyes from excessive fatigue.

Which is worse for eye strain, being nearsighted or farsighted?

There really is no relation between being nearsighted or farsighted and how susceptible you are to eye strain. It's all a matter of how you are using your eyes, under what lighting, for what length of time, and in what environment. Both near and farsighted individuals are equally susceptible to eye strain.

Does eye strain cause "floaters?"

Eye strain does not cause floaters. These tiny specks or spots in our eyes are bits of the vitreous that have broken away. They are most visible when we are looking at a clear, bright surface like the screen of a computer. Floaters are a natural consequence of aging.

Does bright sunlight contribute to eye strain?

Yes, any kind of bright light will make eye strain worse.
When you are outdoors, even on overcast days, you should
always wear tinted lenses that block 100% of UV rays.

**I've never needed glasses but my near vision is suddenly
bad. Why?**

By age 40, the vast majority of people suffer from some
degree of age-related presbyopia. If you have never worn
glasses, go ahead and get an eye exam. It's likely that you
need reading glasses. If you do not require any adjustment
to your vision beyond magnification, you can likely make
use of over-the-counter "readers."

How common is glaucoma?

Estimates suggest that approximately 67 million people
worldwide have glaucoma. It is the second leading cause of
blindness, and thus is one of the most compelling reasons
for people to have an annual eye exam.

What are the risk factors for glaucoma?

The six greatest risk factors for glaucoma are: more than 50
years of age, a history of glaucoma in the family, extreme
nearsightedness, high fluid pressure readings with large
daily fluctuations, thin corneas, being of African descent.

If I have high blood pressure, will the pressure in my eyes also be high?

In older patients there is an indirect relationship between high blood pressure and glaucoma, but patients who are under stress or who experience sudden blood pressure spikes typically do not have a corresponding high fluid pressure in the eyes.

Can glaucoma cause a headache and eye strain?

No, there are no evident signs of glaucoma. You will not experience either a headache or eye strain.

Does eye strain cause cataracts?

No, cataracts, which are a clouding of the lens of the eyes, are typically a consequence of aging. Because the clouding makes it extremely difficult for a person to focus, once the cataracts are even moderately advanced, their presence makes it much easier for the eyes to become fatigued and strained.

What is the relationship between eye strain and migraines?

The two are not directly related. Migraines are caused by a release of inflammatory chemicals deep in the brains of susceptible individuals. Eye strain is caused by over use of the eyes. However, if you are someone with a predisposition for migraines, eye fatigue can bring on an episode, which may include visual symptoms like flashes and auras.

Afterword

Getting a handle on persistent eye strain is not so much a matter of finding a "cure" as it is finding the factors that are contributing to the stress being placed on your eyes and doing something to change or remove them.

For many people, the answer may be as simple as different or better lighting, or just keeping their computer screen cleaner to avoid glare. Simple changes in habit, like sitting the correct distance from the monitor, can make all the difference in the world.

So long as you begin to address your eye strain be getting a comprehensive exam from a qualified eye doctor, there is no reason why you cannot manage your eye fatigue with proven home remedies.

Our eyes are put to task daily in our computer driven, digitally intense, 21st century world. It's no longer just an issue of staring at a monitor too long, but rather the ubiquitous presence of tablets, ereaders, and smartphones that have us squinting at tiny letters on overly bright screens for hours at a time.

Although not dangerous, eye strain is exhausting and will drag down your productivity and your enjoyment of life if you do not identify what's causing the problem and find a solution.

This may mean glasses, or it may mean just forcing yourself to take a break more often. Regardless, once recognized, eye strain is a problem that can not only be managed, but also solved entirely.

Relevant Websites

7 Bad Habits That Are Aging Your Eyes
www.allaboutvision.com/resources/bad-habits.htm

7 Easy Ways to Save Your Eyes from Smartphone Strain
www.entrepreneur.com/article/232665

All About Myopia
www.myeyes.com/myopia/all-about-myopia.shtml

American Optometric Association
www.aoa.org

Astigmatism
www.aoa.org/patients-and-public/eye-and-vision-
problems/glossary-of-eye-and-vision-
conditions/astigmatism?sso=y

Computer Eye Strain: 10 Steps for Relief
www.allaboutvision.com/cvs/irritated.htm

Do E-Readers Cause Eye Strain?
bits.blogs.nytimes.com/2010/02/12/do-e-readers-cause-eye-
strain/?_r=1

E-Readers: Better for Your Eyes?
www.medcan.com/articles/e-readers_better_for_your_eyes/

Eye Fatigue - WebMD
www.webmd.com/eye-health/eye-fatigue-causes-
symptoms-treatment

Eye Floaters and Spots in Your Vision
www.eyedoctorguide.com/eye_problems/eye-floaters.html

Eye Floaters, Flashes and Spots
www.allaboutvision.com/conditions/spotsfloats.htm

Eye Health and Retinal Detachment - WebMD
www.webmd.com/eye-health/eye-health-retinal-detachment?page=2

Eye Strain - Mayo Clinic
www.mayoclinic.org/diseases-conditions/eyestrain/basics/definition/con-20032649

Facts About Cataracts
www.nei.nih.gov/health/cataract/cataract_facts

Farsightedness (Hyperopia)
www.rexburgvision.com/Hyperopia.html

The Glaucoma Foundation
www.glaucomafoundation.org

How to Read Your Eyeglass Prescription
www.allaboutvision.com/eyeglasses/eyeglass-prescription.htm

National Eye Institute
www.nei.nih.gov/

Understanding Presbyopia
www.beaumontvision.com/understanding-presbyopia/

Top 10 Home Remedies to Reduce Eye Strain
naturalcuresnotmedicine.com/top-10-home-remedies-to-reduce-eye-strain/

Glossary

amblyopia - A lazy or wandering eye that does not track appropriately in the socket. This is not the same condition as a ptosis.

aqueous humor - Clear fluid that fills the space between the cornea at the front of the eye and the lens.

asthenopia - The ophthalmological term for the condition commonly referred to as eye strain or eye fatigue.

astigmatism - A defect in the eye that causes a deviation from the structure's spherical curvature with a resulting focal distortion of images transmitted via the retina to the brain.

cataracts - A condition of the eye that causes the lens to become increasingly opaque, resulting in blurred vision.

choroid - The choroid is the eye's vascular layer that contains connective tissue and lies between the retina and the sclera.

computer glasses - Prescription eyewear that has been optimized to focus at the ideal distance for a computer monitor to be positioned 20-24 inches from your eyes

conjunctivitis - Conjunctivitis or pink eye is an inflammation of the thin, clear tissue covering the white part of the eye and the inside of the eyelid. This tissue, called the conjunctiva, may become irritated by the presence of a virus or bacteria, or due to exposure to chemical irritants (chlorine, smoke, shampoo). Allergens such as dust and pollen can also be involved.

constriction - The act of closing, as in "constriction of the pupil" indicating that less light is allowed to enter the eye.

cornea - The clear layer at the front of the eye through which light passes on its way to the lens.

diabetic retinopathy - A complication of diabetes that damages the blood vessels of the retina, which can either be minor in nature or affect a person's ability to see.

dilation - The act of opening, as in "dilation of the pupil" indicating more light is allowed into the eye.

dry eye - A disease of the eye characterized by inadequate tear production necessitating the frequent daily use of lubricating drops.

eyeglasses - Lens designed with specific degrees of curvature to correct visual abnormalities. Lenses may be single vision to correct near or farsightedness, or bifocals (outfitted with two regions to correct near and far vision.) If additional correction is required, with a medium area of adjustment, the lenses are said to be "progressive."

glaucoma - A condition in which pressure in the eyeball increases to abnormal levels and can, if left untreated, cause blindness.

hordeolum - A hordeolum or sty is a painful, red lump that sits at the edge of your eyelid. It has the appearance of a small pimple or boil.

hyperopia - A visual abnormality commonly known as farsightedness that allows a person to only see objects at a distance clearly.

iris - The iris, located behind the cornea, is a flat membrane in the eye shaped like a ring with an adjustable center pupil.

keratometer - A diagnostic instrument that measures the curvature of the front of the eye to determine the extent and axis of astigmatism.

lens - The lens is the transparent structure in the eye that works with the cornea to refract light rays on to the retina.

macular degeneration - An eye disease that causes a gradual loss of vision over time, although rarely does the affected person go completely blind. Primarily the central portion of the field of vision is affected.

myopia - A visual abnormality commonly known as nearsightedness that allows a person to only see objects that are close at hand.

ocular - Of or pertaining to the eye and vision.

ocular migraine - An ocular migraine is caused by the same release of inflammatory chemicals deep in the brain as a regular migraine, but there is no pain. Instead, a blind spot develops in the center of the field of vision surrounded by pulsating, wavy, colored lines. The phenomenon lasts approximately 30 minutes, and is not dangerous.

ophthalmologist - A professional who holds a degree as either a Doctor of Osteopathy or a Doctor of Medicine. They provide comprehensive eye care including diagnosing and treating common and complex eye problems, performing eye surgeries, and prescribing corrective lenses.

optician - A specialist trained to assemble, fit, and sell prescription eyeglasses and, in some areas, contact lenses.

optic nerve - Each of two optic nerves sits at the back of the retina to receive nerve impulses for transmission to the brain where those impulses are assembled as a visual image.

optometrists - A professional who holds a degree in optometry and carries the title doctor. Their purpose is to evaluate vision, diagnose general eye conditions, and prescribe corrective lenses.

pachymetry - A process to measure the thickness of the human cornea.

peripheral vision - The degree to which a person can see on either side of their head while keeping their eyes focused forward.

perimetry - Taking the measurement of the width of a person's field of vision.

phoropter - An ophthalmic testing device containing different lenses used during sight testing to refine a prescription. Also called a refractor.

photophobia - Severe sensitivity to light that causes discomfort and pain even indoors. People with light colored eyes are more susceptible.

presbyopia - A condition that begins after the age of 40 when vision becomes blurred for tasks near at hand as a natural consequence of aging.

pupil - The pupil is the adjustable circular opening in the center of the iris which dilates and constricts to control the amount of light entering the eye.

ptosis - A ptosis is an upper or lower eyelid that droops because the muscles that raise the eyelid are abnormally weak. Some individuals are born with the condition, while others experience the drooping as they age or as a symptom of another illness.

retina - The retina is a layer at the back of the eye that contains light sensitive cells that trigger nerve impulses transmitted via the optic nerve to the brain where a visual image is formed.

sclera - The white outer layer of the eye, which, with the cornea, forms the external covering of the eyeball.

scotoma - A blind spot in the field of vision, like the temporary pulsating, multi-colored patches that appear during an ocular migraine.

sty - A sty or hordeolum is a painful, red lump that sits at the edge of your eyelid. It has the appearance of a small pimple or boil.

tonometer - A tonometer is an instrument used to measure the pressure of the eyeball to determine if glaucoma is present.

Index

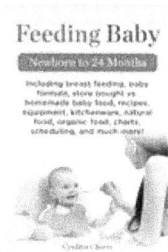

Feeding Baby
Cynthia Cherry
978-1941070000

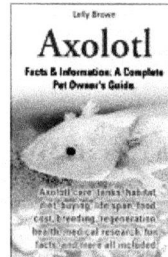

Axolotl
Lolly Brown
978-0989658430

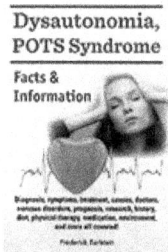

Dysautonomia, POTS
Syndrome
Frederick Earlstein
978-0989658485

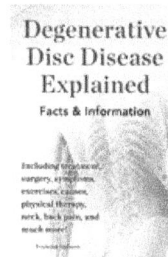

Degenerative Disc
Disease Explained
Frederick Earlstein
978-0989658485

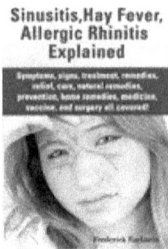

Sinusitis, Hay Fever,
Allergic Rhinitis Explained
Frederick Earlstein
978-1941070024

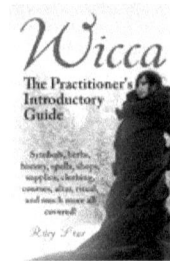

Wicca
Riley Star
978-1941070130

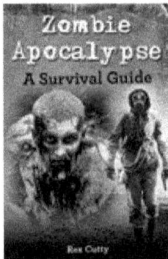

Zombie Apocalypse
Rex Cutty
978-1941070154

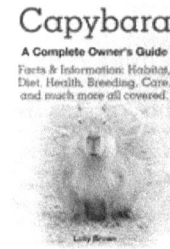

Capybara
Lolly Brown
978-1941070062

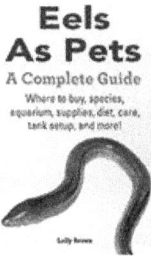

Eels As Pets
Lolly Brown
978-1941070167

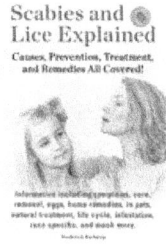

Scabies and Lice Explained
Frederick Earlstein
978-1941070017

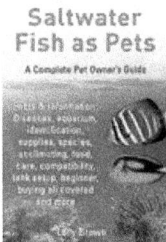

Saltwater Fish As Pets
Lolly Brown
978-0989658461

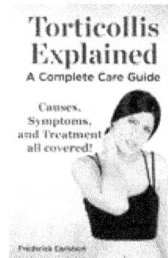

Torticollis Explained
Frederick Earlstein
978-1941070055

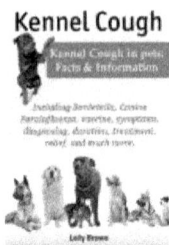

Kennel Cough
Lolly Brown
978-0989658409

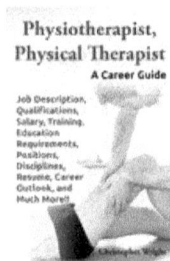

Physiotherapist, Physical
Therapist
Christopher Wright
978-0989658492

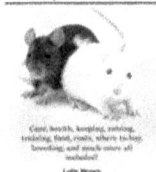

Rats, Mice, and Dormice
As Pets
Lolly Brown
978-1941070079

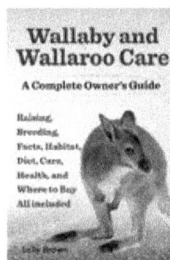

Wallaby and Wallaroo Care
Lolly Brown
978-1941070031

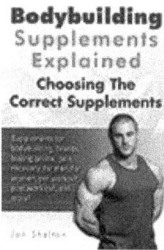

Bodybuilding Supplements
Explained
Jon Shelton
978-1941070239

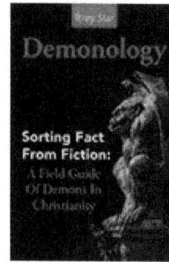

Demonology
Riley Star
978-19401070314

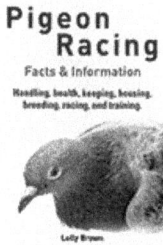

Pigeon Racing
Lolly Brown
978-1941070307

www.ingramcontent.com/pod-product-compliance
Lightning Source LLC
Chambersburg PA
CBHW060640210326
41520CB00010B/1673